Hypertrophy – The Science of Building Muscle

I0407377

Discover the Secrets to Muscle Growth, Supreme Strength and Maintaining a Healthy Diet

RON KNESS

Contents

Disclaimer

This publication is for informational purposes only and is not intended as medical advice. Medical advice should always be obtained from a qualified medical professional for any health conditions or symptoms associated with them.

Every possible effort has been made in preparing and researching this material. We make no warranties with respect to the accuracy, applicability of its contents or any omissions.

See your healthcare professional before starting any diet or exercise program!

Introduction

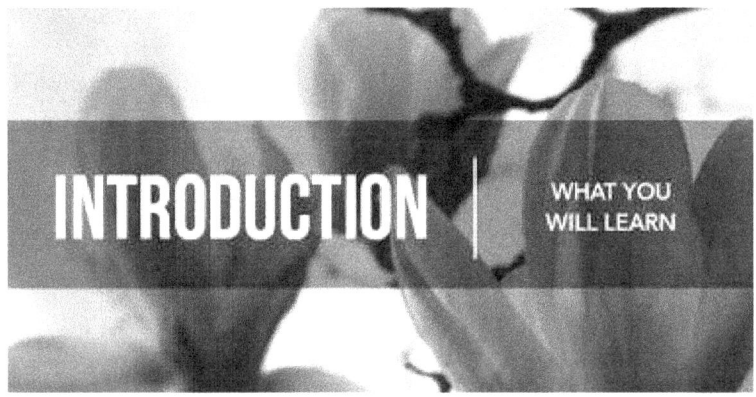

Building muscle is at once very simple and simultaneously incredibly complicated. If that sounds like something of a frustrating contradiction… well then get used to it! As you learn more about growing muscle and getting jacked, you'll find that almost all the information you come across only makes things more complicated and more difficult. Everyone has a different opinion and no-one seems able to agree on what the best way to get into powerful shape actually is.

When you start out though, it all seems very straightforward. In order to grow, you need to exercise more and eat more protein. When you do this, you start to build more muscle and you'll see yourself constantly increase in strength. If you aren't seeing any growth or strength gains, then it might well simply mean you aren't going to the gym regularly enough, or working out hard enough when you are there!

And for the most part, this is fairly accurate. No matter what kind of training you are using, lifting weight and eating more meat should result in some muscle mass. Overcomplicating things at this stage will only make it harder to stay motivated and result in poor results.

But over time, you start to notice that you aren't seeing change as quickly as you'd like. You realize that your colleagues-in-iron are getting results faster than you and that you've 'plateaued', whatever that might mean. That's when you start to read into training and learn that there's more than one way to skin a cat.

This is when you learn the best way to build muscle is to lift heavy and for fewer reps. You need to focus on compound lifts so your strength gains are "functional" and you should support that with a healthy, ketogenic diet.

But then there's another guy who's saying something really rather different. This guy reckons you should isolate your muscles during training and focus on just the one muscle group to cause the maximum muscle damage in the way of micro-tears. And while you're at it, you need to focus on higher rep ranges because really, the only thing that matters is "time under tension".

Then someone comes over to you in the gym and corrects your technique – even though you learned it on YouTube – and you find yourself just about ready to give up on the whole thing. Training is just too complicated!

The Different Types of Muscle

What you're experiencing here is the classic problem: "a little bit of knowledge is a very dangerous thing". Unfortunately, everyone on the internet thinks they're an expert and they're very ready to tell you what the best way to build muscle is based on a very small amount of reading and very limited experience of their own.

But if you can spend enough time learning the whole picture, you'll realize that there is no right way to build muscle and there is no wrong way. The reality is there are different body types and there are different goals. The type of training you use should be based on the type of body you have and what you respond well to, as well as the type of training that most interests you and the goals that you're looking to accomplish.

This isn't just something people say, it's 100% true.

Once you know what your body responds to, once you know what your goals are and once you understand how hypertrophy (muscle growth) works; then you can pick the very best muscle building strategy that will help you to see the most growth the most quickly. Once you find this ideal combination, your gains will completely accelerate and you'll see much more impressive gains than you ever have done before.

And guess what? That's just what we're going to learn in this book. We're going to learn the science behind muscle growth and strength gains and we're going to discover the different ways to progress in each area. By the end, you'll understand the differences between bodybuilding, powerlifting and power building. You'll learn some very surprising ways to quickly gain a LOT of muscle and you'll experience some highly efficient and punishing training methods that are quite unlike anything you've seen before.

To summarize, you'll discover:

- The difference between fast and slow twitch muscle fiber

- The difference between "sarcoplasmic" and "myofibrillar" hypertrophy

- How to combine different types of training to experience "athletic aesthetics"

- Why both compound AND isolation movements are perfectly valid

- How to train faster for better results

- How to use the Joe Weider intensity principles

- How to see growth even as a "hard gainer"

- How to become incredibly lean and ripped, even as an endomorph

- How to work out your "training philosophy"

- How to choose a fitness movement that works for you

- How to develop a training program and stick to it

- And much more!

The Types of Hypertrophy

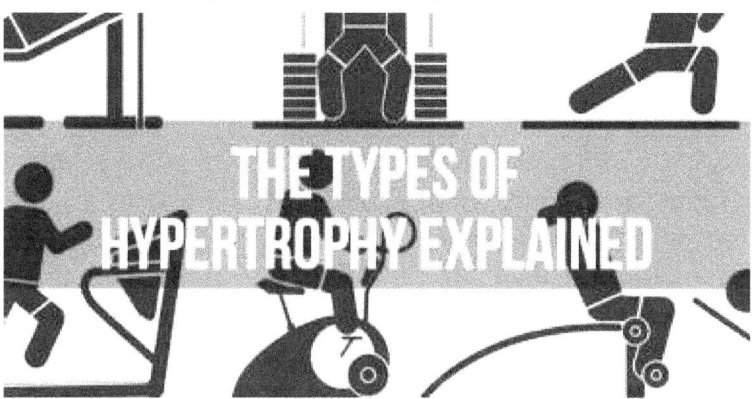

Let's start at the beginning, with the different types of hypertrophy and how each of them can be employed to get different results.

Actually, let's rewind and start even further at the beginning. Specifically, let's take a look at why you need to know why you're training before you even begin.

You see, the way you're going to train is always going to be dictated by the results that you're looking for. This might sound obvious but actually it's something that a lot of people never consider before they start working out. They just say they want to be "fitter". That term can mean different things to different people.

But the real question is "What does fitter meant to you?" Is it strong with lots of bulky muscle? Or is it strong without muscle? Or is it in a much leaner sense? Or is it something in between?

Why is it you train? Is it because you want to be a kind of super hero? In that case, you'll be well suited to a GPP system like CrossFit.

This stands for "General Physical Preparedness" and basically means you're strong and fit across the board and thereby able to defend yourself during a zombie apocalypse.

Maybe you're an amateur athlete and you want to be particularly impressive in a specific domain as a runner, in long jump, or in some other context.

Or maybe you just want to be a little fitter and healthier so you can be a good influence for your children and be a more active and engaged parent. And maybe you'd just like to wake up full of energy for a change and try to avoid getting colds quite so frequently.

Whatever the case – in all these scenarios - the type of training you're going to do is going to be completely different. And that's before we've even acknowledged the significant difference between different body types. Because what helps one person to quickly build a huge amount of muscle just won't work for the next guy.

How can you know what is the best way to train unless you know these things? How can you expect to be met with anything other than frustration if you don't know what it is you're hoping to achieve?

Ultimately, having a goal is a little bit like knowing what your destination is. Knowing your body type, is like knowing what kind of gas your car likes. Without these crucial bits of information, you really can't expect to reach your destination (goal) very quickly (if at all)!

How Hypertrophy Works

So with all that in mind, you should be going into this chapter with a good idea of what it is you want to accomplish. Only that way, will you be able to take the relevant information from this and ignore all the rest.

So what is hypertrophy? When your muscles grow, what actually causes them to grow? What is actually happening? As you probably had already guessed, there's actually multiple things going on, which is where all the confusion comes in.

Generally though, we can split hypertrophy down into two main processes. These are "sarcoplasmic" and "myofibrillar" hypertrophy. Actually though, even this is contested somewhat – some experts actually believe these terms are merely pseudoscience and that they aren't actually based on any concrete evidence.

But whether or not the precise principles of hypertrophy are accurate or not, the reality is that these two types of training do result in two different types of muscle. This is how strength athletes have been training for decades, with a lot of success, so it's safe for us to take this understanding and apply it. These terms and the description will simply serve as a somewhat useful "crutch" for understanding what's going on here…

Myofibrillar Hypertrophy

So on the one hand, we have myofibrillar hypertrophy, which is the predominant form of hypertrophy used for building strength. This is also sometimes referred to more simply as "muscle damage".

And that's an apt name because it really does describe what is going on here – you are damaging the muscle.

Or more specifically, you're actually tearing the muscle. By lifting heavy enough weights, you're actually causing tiny rips in the fibers that make up the muscle, known as muscle fibers (the tears themselves are called "micro tears").

Muscle fibers work just like any other cell in the human body, except that they can have multiple mitochondria and can also increase as you train more frequently and in higher volumes. Right now though, we're interested in tearing the muscle fiber, which then causes it to be marked for repair. Once we're sleeping or resting, these tears are then repaired by the body using protein and amino acids to restore the muscle and build the muscle fibers to be thicker and stronger.

It's generally agreed that it's impossible to increase the number of muscle fibers (a process that is known as hyperplasia) through conventional training. However, you can increase the thickness of the fibers through this process which makes them stronger and increases your ability to throw heavy weights around.

What's the best way to cause these micro tears? That would be to train with heavier weights, which in turn will allow you to cause more damage more quickly, triggering more growth. That's why powerlifters – who are predominantly interested in pure power – will train using weights close to their one rep maxes and lift only a few times.

Sarcoplasmic Hypertrophy

Then you have sarcoplasmic hypertrophy, which is also sometimes known as "metabolic stress". Here, the objective is not to create micro tears but rather to swell the muscles with metabolites, metabolites being hormones and other compounds that stimulate more growth and hypertrophy. The obvious examples of these are testosterone and growth hormone, both of which are anabolic in nature.

So how do you trigger this kind of change in your body? This time, the aim is to occlude the muscle and allow blood to build up there – right up until the point where you have too much lactic acid in your muscles to continue and you start to feel a lot of discomfort. You do this by using higher repetitions, as this allows you to increase that all-important "time under tension" – the amount of time that your muscle spends contracting during any given workout.

While the precise mechanism of action isn't fully understood, this appears to increase the amount of sarcoplasm in the muscle cells – their ability to retain fluid and to store glycogen. This in turn then allows the lifter to continue lifting for longer and to see more growth.

While myofibrillar hypertrophy does lead to some increase in size as well as strength, sarcoplasmic hypertrophy appears to be the fastest way to increase size. A bodybuilder trains with significantly lighter weights but uses higher rep ranges, often reaching into the 10s, 12s and 15s before they reach failure.

This is why a considerably smaller powerlifter will often be able to lift more than a much larger bodybuilder. But that is not to say that a bodybuilder's muscle isn't as "strong" or that one type of lifting is better than the other.

We're going to get into all that in MUCH more detail over the subsequent chapters.

Understanding the Types of Hypertrophy

For now though, a quick takeaway…

- To build more SIZE and less strength, you need to lift lighter weights for longer periods of time.

- To build more STRENGTH and less size, you need to lift very heavy weights for fewer repetitions.

You can also tell which type of muscle you're building based on the way your body feels at the time – and this is something you might get better at differentiating between as you progress. Myofibrillar hypertrophy feels like tearing at the time (not a serious tear however) and leads to DOMS (delayed onset muscle soreness) the next day or the day after.

Conversely, sarcoplasmic hypertrophy is what leads to the feeling of the 'pump' as you train and your muscles become massively swelled with muscle. It's also what eventually leads to "the burn" talked about as the muscle floods with lactic acid, resulting in a lot of discomfort. This is where expressions like "no pain, no gain" come from!

Training for Power, Functional Strength with High Weight

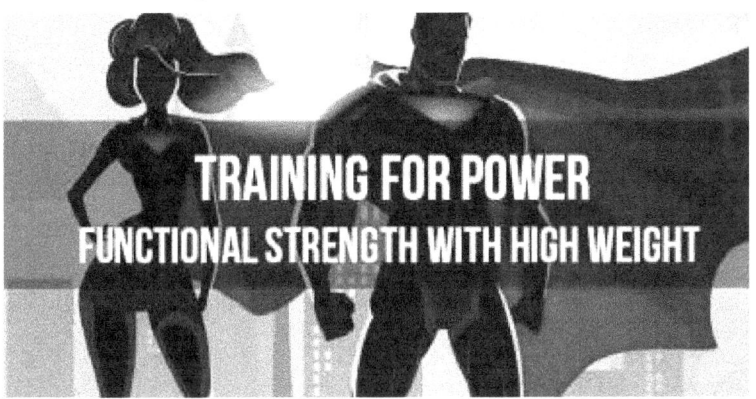

So now you understand those differences, you're starting to get an idea of how you train for strength and power: you use heavier weights and you perform fewer repetitions to create lots of micro tears.

But this…

…is to go…

…even further…

…BEYOND!

Because actually, there's a lot more to it than that!

Functional Strength

The first thing to consider is that lifting for pure power will always need to involve training for functional strength primarily.

In turn, this means that you're lifting very heavy weights through larger ranges of motion that incorporate lots of muscles into one clean and smooth movement. Examples of "compound" lifts include the squat, the deadlift and the bench press. In each case, all the muscles are working together in unison in order to drive the weight. This means you're using your legs, your core, your lower back and your arms all at the same time and it means that technique is going to be much more important.

These moves are called functional because they mimic the way that you use your body in the real world. In real life, we very rarely use any movements that only utilize one muscle group on its own. When you perform a bicep curl, you'll move the weight through a set range of motion and the only pivot point will be your elbow. There are very few scenarios quite like this outside of the gym.

Conversely, performing a deadlift means coordinating your whole body, which is also what happens when you push your sofa during redecorating, when you wrestle and when you open the garage door. Therefore, it is considered more functional.

These kinds of compound, functional movements are also favored by many people thanks to their ability to stimulate more anabolic compounds. Deadlifting and squatting both result in the release of more growth hormone and more testosterone and the simple reason for this is that they incorporate more muscles and more of the larger muscles.

This is true to the point that some people claim you can't build big muscle without using compound movements. This isn't true as we'll see... but certainly compound lifts are great for inciting more growth.

Muscle Fiber Types

There's another factor to consider when lifting very heavy weights and another reason that you need the heaviest weights in order to stimulate the most strength.

And this has to do with "fast twitch" and "slow twitch" muscle fiber types.

Fast twitch muscle fibers are the muscle fibers that we use for explosive movements. These rely on glycogen stored in the muscles in order to operate and they are capable of exerting much more force compared with slow twitch fibers. At the same time though, fast twitch muscle fibers also wear out faster and aren't as energy efficient. A long distance runner then will have more slow twitch muscle fiber, while a powerlifter or a sprinter will have more fast twitch muscle fiber.

Anatomically, this is because fast twitch muscle fibers have more stored glycogen and fewer mitochondria. Mitochondria are what convert glucose into ATP which is energy used by the cell using the aerobic system. Conversely, glycogen is available for immediate use, though stores are depleted very quickly.

The body will always use the most efficient combination of muscle fibers possible to get the job done. You can't half use a muscle fiber, they are binary in nature. That means each muscle fiber either kicks in, or it doesn't, kind of like a digital signal verses an analog if you are familiar with electronics.

If you lift something light then, your body will likely use a couple of fast twitch fibers but a lot more slow twitch muscle.

This will allow you to curl for longer, but it means you won't be tearing/stimulating the fast twitch fibers that give you that maximum strength.

Conversely, when you lift something very heavy, the muscles will be forced to recruit more fast twitch muscle fiber just to shift that weight. Therefore, you'll eventually tear the fast twitch fibers, thus resulting in the stimulation you need to trigger growth. So you really do need to lift heavy in order to engage the fast twitch muscle fibers.

Individual Differences

This is where individual differences start to come into play though. Because actually, some people have more fast twitch muscle fiber genetically, while others have more slow twitch. This immediately impacts on the type of training they are going to respond best to. People with more fast twitch muscle fiber might be particularly adept at lifting heavy weights for fewer repetitions and might find this leads to rapid hypertrophy. On the other hand, those who have a lot more slow twitch fiber, will often find that they actually respond a lot better when they lighten their load and start lifting lighter weights for more repetitions!

The Role of the Central Nervous System

Also very important to understand is the role of the central nervous system and the brain.

And this is how someone like Bruce Lee was capable of doing incredible things like holding a 40kg barbell at arm's length.

Because in order to utilize your muscle at any point, you first need to send the relevant signals from your brain. Those signals then need to travel through your central nervous system and reach the muscles by crossing the point called the 'neuromuscular junction'. When they reach this point, a signal is sent across using the chemical acetylcholine and a small electrical impulse called an action potential. When that signal is strong enough, it is able to cause the fibers it comes into contact with to fire, which in turn makes the muscles lift the weight.

If the signal isn't strong enough, then a lower proportion of the muscle fibers will fire – even though you might need to engage more of them to lift the weight.

What does this tell us? It tells us that the brain might just be the bottleneck in some cases, not the muscle itself.

And actually, this is always the case. When you attempt to lift a truly heavy weight, you'll find that the most you can possibly recruit – even as a trained athlete – is up to 50% of your muscle fiber.

And if you're not a trained athlete? Then you're looking at much closer to 30% in most cases.

So with the best will in the world, you're only going to be able to engage up to 50% of your maximum strength at any one time! And this strength is also going to be highly dependent on your tiredness and other factors.

At this point, you might be wondering why muscle fiber recruitment is so low. Why wouldn't we be able to engage all our muscle in one go?

But the answer comes down to evolution. In the wild, if we were to engage 100% of our fast twitch muscle fiber to the point that it fatigued, then we'd be left with zero energy left to engage. As a result, we'd then be completely spent if we were to need that muscle later on. Imagine if you saw a predator and you had completely exhausted all of your muscle power! Imagine not even being able to crawl to find food!

And then there's the very distinct possibility that you could end up causing injury to yourself without any limit on your strength. You'd probably end up dislocating your own joints every time you moved!

And thus, we can only engage a proportion of our muscle mass unless….

The Mind Muscle Connection

Simply by training with the heaviest weights possible, you are going to find that you immediately increase your "mind-muscle connection". That's because you're going to be at least trying to engage as much muscle as possible. And the law of SAID (Specific Adaptations to Imposed Demands) tells us this would then make us better at recruiting that muscle in future.

But you can also engage muscle fiber in some other ways. One method is to use something called overbearing isometrics. An isometric exercise is anything that involves contracting the muscle without moving it – a "static hold". Normally, this means holding a weight until you can't hold it anymore and you slowly let it drop.

When your aim is to increase the mind muscle connection though, you can do this another way by pulling or pushing against an immovable force. Bruce Lee used to do this by chaining a barbell to the floor and then trying to squat or curl it. This is the equivalent of trying to lift 100% of your 1 rep maximum (the most weight you can move for one repetition) and as far as your body is concerned, there is zero difference!

Another way to build the mind-muscle connection is to practice contracting the muscle and really focusing on it – both during exercises and immediately after. If you watch strength athletes on YouTube, they'll often contract their muscles and pull a pose straight after lifting. That's not (just) vanity – it's also to help enforce that connection.

This is also why it's so important not to just let your mind wander during your training, but to focus on what you are doing.

Hysterical Strength

If you wanted to go beyond even powerlifting-strength and see what it's like to experience the kind of strength that's almost superhuman, then you may be interested in stories demonstrating hysterical strength.

Hysterical strength is a term that describes the superhuman strength some people experience when they are in extreme danger. When you hear stories of mothers lifting cars off of their children, that's an example of hysterical strength. Another famous story involves a rock climber lifting a rock off of themselves in excess of 300KG.

How is this possible? Well, while these are just urban myths, studies suggest that the right neurochemistry can in fact allow us to override the "safety switch" in our brain and tap into untold power – recruiting up to 100% of our muscle mass. Studies show that adrenaline plays a role in this and that simply tricks like shouting during lifting can create a slight surge in this to allow you to lift heavier.

Of course this is kind of annoying for everyone else in the gym though.

Practice Makes Perfect

Note that the mind-muscle connection is also what we refer to as technique. When you have good technique, it's because you have strengthened connections in the brain corresponding to very precise and specific movements in the body. You're constantly using particular neural networks in your motor cortex and this is in turn going to strengthen those connections and help you to better control your body when performing those precise movements. Not only will this result in better muscle fiber recruitment but it will also help you to more effectively perform the technique, thereby avoiding any wasted energy that might come from overbalancing or otherwise just not performing as well as you might.

Training for Size, Time Under Tension and Slow Eccentrics

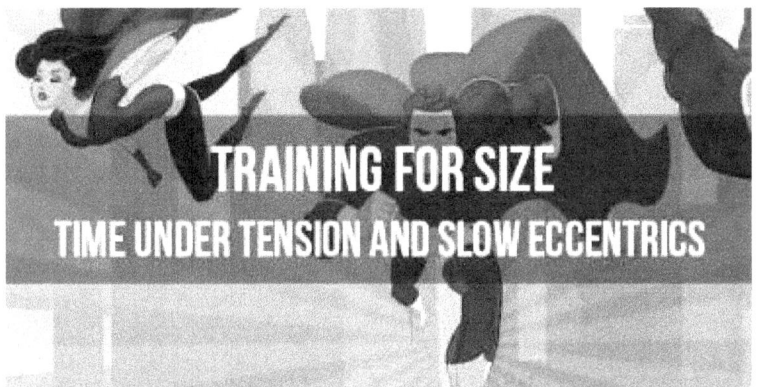

So that last chapter was a very in depth look at how you train for pure strength.

Now it's time to look at how you train for maximum size. What do you need to do to grow above all else?

The answer, as we've seen, lies with time under tension. The more time you spend under tension, the more you allow those all-important metabolites to build up and the more you're going to grow.

This is what will result in the slightly softer, slightly more "bloated" muscle look that you associate with a bodybuilder versus the rock hard, but slightly thinner muscle of a martial artist which is just full of fast-twitch fiber and under tight mental control.

Now here's the myth that we want to dispel right away: bodybuilding muscle is not "fake" muscle. And bodybuilding muscle is in no way 'less functional' than power building muscle.

Remember: this simply comes down to SAID. Yes, power builders are stronger than bodybuilders when it comes to 1RM – the amount of weight lifted for 1 repetition. But a bodybuilder conversely will normally have great muscle endurance. That means they'll be better at continuing to exert force over a longer time – i.e. over more repetitions of the same exercise at the same weight. And this is in no way less important or less impressive than being able to generate explosive force in the short term.

Think about it: in the real world, are you more likely to need to lift something very heavy just once, or are you more likely to need to lift something moderately heavy over and over again? For most of us, the answer is definitely the latter – and this is what bodybuilding muscle provides you with by giving you more glycogen in the muscle.

Time Under Tension

So the objective here is to challenge the muscle to continue to exert itself to the point where it starts to fail from both muscle damage and a buildup of lactic acid (which is a byproduct of the glycogen muscle system).

To really increase time under tension though, we're not only interested in curling weights for longer sets, we're also interested in manipulating our technique such that it will increase the time we spend contracting.

This means, for instance, that you'll be curling the weight without ever quite putting it completely down. You'll be stopping just short of fully locking out the arm and you'll be stopping just short of moving the weight all the weight to the top.

Another way to increase time under tension is simply to slow down your repetitions. By slowing the repetitions down more, you spend more time contracting and you also force better technique, more concentration and great muscle fiber recruitment.

Note that this type of weight lifting still needs to create muscle damage. You still need to progress and that means you're still aiming to create some micro tears. This is where elaborate intensity techniques come in, which involve doing things like curling or pressing very heavy weight, only to then drop immediately to a slightly lower weight (drop set). We'll discuss all this more in a subsequent chapter.

Isolation Exercise

While pure powerlifters will always prefer compound movements, bodybuilders will be much more likely to incorporate isolation movements into their training.

Of course an isolation movement is the opposite of a compound movement. Whereas compound movements involve lifting weights using multiple muscle groups and lots of coordination, isolation movements involve focusing on just the one muscle and making sure not to involve any other muscles at all.

So a bodybuilder will be much more likely to use a bicep curl versus a powerlifter. And the reason for this is that a curl is a single-joint exercise. This only involves one joint in the body and that in turn means that you aren't having to coordinate lots of different muscle groups at once.

But what it also means is that you can really focus on just that one muscle, you can actually cause more micro tears and you can build up more metabolites in that one area.

The problem with using lots of muscles in unison, is that you won't actually be focusing on any one group. When you deadlift, you are using your calves, hamstrings, glutes, quads, core, erector spinae, traps, forearms, shoulders and lats. As soon as the combined strength your muscles are capable of generating meets its limit, you'll not be able to perform any more repetitions. Often it ends up being the forearms that let the team down!

Conversely, with a curl, you are pretty much only focusing on the biceps. That means you can keep going until the biceps give up.

What's more, is that you can much more safely keep pushing yourself when you're using an isolation movement. With a squat, piling on more and more weight and performing more and more repetitions will eventually cause your form to suffer as key muscles start to struggle. If you keep going beyond that point, you can then injure your back or your knee. With a single-joint exercise on the other hand, you can keep going until the weight literally drops out of your hand. That means you can train for much more muscle damage and much more metabolic stress in that specific region.

The way a bodybuilder will often train then, is to use isolation exercises that repeatedly focus on the same muscle and repeatedly fatigue it.

They cause so much muscle damage and metabolic stress that it takes several days for the muscles to recover and become useable again – but in the meantime they'll focus on training other body parts on different days.

Negatives and Eccentric Isometrics

Bodybuilders that are purely interested in size do have something in common with powerlifters though – that being their love of the fast twitch muscle fiber.

This is because fast twitch muscle fiber just so happens to be thicker and therefore larger looking than slow twitch muscle fiber (which is why endurance athletes tend to look very lean). A bodybuilder looking to build strength then would be interested in causing muscle damage to the fast twitch fiber, which is why they still need to use weights that are in their 8-10 rep max, rather than curling for 20 or 30 repetitions.

This is also why a bodybuilder might place more emphasis on the eccentric portions of their movements. So what is that? It's essentially the aim to create more muscle tears, without necessarily having to lift massive weights for just a few repetitions.

Muscle fiber just so happens to be strongest in the negative, eccentric portion of the movement. That means it is stronger when the muscle is contracting, meaning that you can hold a heavier weight than you can lift.

Thus, when you lift a heavy weight and lower it very slowly, you will be able to cause more damage to the fast twitch muscle fiber.

Many bodybuilders then incorporate eccentric isometrics (or quasi-isometrics) by very slowly lowering the weight for the count of 2-7 seconds. This also increases time under tension in the most efficient way and in general can stimulate a lot of growth.

This is another reason bodybuilders will use lighter weights – because it allows them to use more controlled technique like this and thereby trigger more tears, more damage and in the end, more growth.

Powerbuilding and Cardio for Supreme Strength

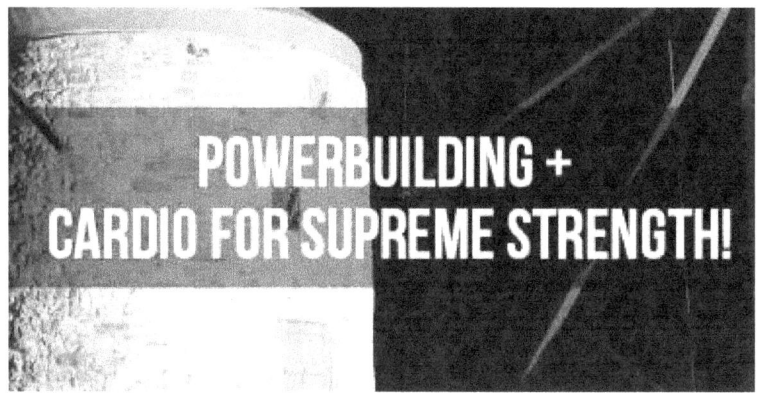

So with all of that in mind, what is the very best way to go about triggering hypertrophy?

Well, as you can see – it very much depends on your muscle and your goals. If you only care about strength, then you need to lift very heavy weights and use explosive movements. You'll want to use functional movements explained earlier that involve lots of compound, multi-joint exercises. You'll also need to focus on your mind muscle connection and your technique. If you only care about size though, then you'll probably use more isolation movements and you'll likely combine that with higher rep ranges but lower weights, designed to flood the muscles with metabolites that will trigger growth via sarcoplasmic hypertrophy. You might also use slower eccentric portions of each move in order to further cause the right kind of muscle damage that will stimulate growth.

But what if you don't have to choose? What if you can train for both size and strength at the same time?

And what if this was actually the most effective way to accomplish both of those things?

This is where power building comes in and actually, it's possibly the best approach you can take to your training unless you're a competitive athlete.

What is Power building?

So what is power building? Simply, it means that you're training half for size and half for strength and thereby using both types of training method to trigger both types of result. You'll be lifting heavier weights, while at the same time also using higher rep ranges.

This is going to actually trigger the most strength and size compared with any other training methodology. For starters, when you combine both types of training, it simply means that you are going to get both kinds of results. That effectively means your results can double up and when you combine both, you see even more impressive growth.

In other words, why would you only thicken your muscle fibers or only swell your muscle with sarcoplasm when you can actually do both? Why would you only train your fast twitch muscle fiber, or only train your slow twitch muscle fiber when once again... you can do both!

Likewise, it makes a lot of sense to use this kind of approach when you aren't sure what kind of training your body is going to respond best to. Because while you might not think you're someone who can build muscle, the reality is that you probably are – you're just not doing it in the most efficient way.

If you normally train with heavy weights and low volume, then you may notice that you hit a plateau and your muscles stop growing. What many people find is that when they use lighter weights and really slow down their repetitions, this is then what results in a sudden increase in gains.

Conversely though, other people find the exact opposite thing: they find when they increase the weight and even when they increase the speed, this triggers the biggest changes. This might be to do with their ratio of fast twitch to slow twitch muscle fibers, or it might be to do with their metabolic makeup and their hormones. Either way, the only way to find out what is going to work (or work best) is to try every method. When you combine multiple types of training into one routine – such as power building – that is exactly what you are doing. If you are using every type of training, then you are going to see results across the board.

And of course this will also result in strength that is in truth the most functional. Because sometimes it's functional to have great explosive strength. Other times it's functional to have great muscle endurance…

So why not just combine both and by doing so, you really maximize your potential and accomplish that general preparedness.

How This Looks in Practice

So that's the theory and principle behind power building, but what does it look like in practice? How can you really combine these two very different training modalities into one form of training? How can you train for two different things at once?

That actually depends and there are a lot of different ways people go about this. One answer people use is to train using one modality on one day and then to train using another modality o another day. So for instance, this might mean that their training regime includes a traditional bodybuilding split for focusing on each major muscle group but that it then also includes a couple of days dedicated to more traditional powerlifting training with the big lifts.

Another option is to use compound moves at the start of a workout and then to use lighter weights and isolation movements toward the end. This way, you can recruit maximum strength for your big lifts right at the start and then fatigue the individual muscles at the end afterward. This will work even better too, because you'll have pre-exhausted the muscle prior to going into that training. This therefore means that the muscle you're focusing on will be much easier to damage and much quicker to respond to an isolation routine.

Drop Sets – The Secret to Incredible Size AND Power

Or you can go one step further and combine powerlifting and bodybuilding methods into single sets. The way you might do this is with a drop set or giant set.

A drop set simply means you are consistently lowering the weight in order to go past failure. Often in bodybuilding, this will take the form of "running the rack".

Here, a weightlifter will start with a heavy weight that they can lift using their chosen exercise for about 8 reps. They will keep lifting until they reach the point of failure, then they'll simply put those weights down and pick up the next lowest from the dumbbell rack.

They then repeat this again and again and again as they move further down the rack to lower weights. Each time though, they are starting from failure on the previous set of exercises, meaning that even very light weights will pose a challenge.

This technique is used in bodybuilding largely because it allows the lifter to increase their time under tension by starting with heavier weights and gradually progressing downward with lighter weights.

But you can actually take this concept even further by using a much heavier lift. Here, you might start with your 3RM (three rep max – the maximum amount of weight you can lift for only three times) as your starting weight and then drop down from there to something slightly lower and keep going.

Now what's happening? Simply, you are pushing yourself as hard as you can go by using the most challenging weight available to you. This is going to do all that stuff we talked about to increase strength – recruiting the fast twitch muscle, creating micro tears and strengthening the mind muscle connection over the neuromuscular junction.

But then, instead of stopping as you normally would, you keep going. Now you're entering into maximum time-under-tension territory because you're not giving the muscle a chance to rest but rather, you're flooding it with blood and metabolites. And then you do it again and again.

And actually, this technique will help you to recruit even more fast twitch muscle fiber than simple power lifting. That's because new muscle fibers will need to kick in each time you tear and fatigue the previous ones. So to start with, you recruit as many fast twitch fibers as you can to lift the weight.

Then you reach failure and can't do any more, but you keep going. So on the lower weight, your body now needs to find more muscle fiber to continue doing its job. Thus it's going to recruit more of those slower twitch fibers and any remaining fast twitch fibers. And when they give out, it's going to look for even more.

Keep this process going until you've exhausted nearly everything you've got and cannot lift even the lightest weight!

Then Add Cardiovascular Exercise (CV)!

And then, on top of all this, you're also going to add CV. Or at least, that's my advice.

Why? Because once again, we don't have to choose between functions here. The body abides to the rule of SAID and if you combine cardio challenges with strength challenges, then it will become strong and fit – which is of course beneficial.

Now a lot of people are moving away from steady-state cardio at the moment and preaching the benefits of HIIT. The claim is that steady state cardio isn't good for anything except breaking down muscle, tiring you out and taking much longer to burn less fat.

But the people saying this are those same people who don't understand that bodybuilding muscle isn't fake muscle. Actually, using CV still has some very useful advantages and you should still incorporate it into your training in a big way.

Let's quickly look at the difference between CV and HIIT, look at the history and assess why this is a useful type of training for a power building-type workout.

HIIT vs CV

Traditionally, CV meant going for a run for an hour, using an elliptical machine, or generally just exerting yourself for a long period of time at an intensity that you're capable of maintaining.

The idea was that this form of exercise would keep you in the "fat burning zone". This is 70 beats per minute (BPM) because at that speed, the heart is still able to keep up and provide energy to the muscles from the fat stores. Go faster than this though and you reach the "anaerobic threshold", meaning your body now doesn't have time to burn fat for energy and can only rely on glycogen stores, blood sugar and ATP in the muscles.

Seeing as we want to burn fat, maintaining continuous exertion at 70BPM seems to make sense.

Then came HIIT. This is High Intensity Interval Training and the idea was to exert yourself to a massive degree for a short period. That would mean running or even sprinting for 1 minute and then recovering by jogging slowly for 2 minutes before starting again.

Now you are alternating between aerobic and anaerobic energy. This means you're testing both energy systems in the body and forcing your body to create more mitochondria and to become more energy efficient. What's more, you're using up all the blood sugar and glycogen during the anaerobic periods, thereby forcing your body to look for energy elsewhere the rest of the time. This causes what's known as the "afterburn effect", where the body has to run on fat for a long time after your training because of all the sugar it has burned already.

Although steady state cardio burns more fat in the short term, research found that HIIT would lead to more fat loss in the long term. And what's more, it doesn't take as long seeing as you're pushing yourself so hard.

But before you get carried away and throw out steady state cardio, consider a few factors.

The first is steady-state cardio is good for your heart. Really good in fact. Only steady state cardio (not HIIT) is able to increase the size of the left ventricle in the heart. In turn, this makes it more effective at pumping large amounts of blood around your body and therefore means it doesn't have to pump as fast. In other words, this is how you can lower your resting heart rate so that your body is better at resting and your heart rate staying down when you're not training.

And as we're going to see in a moment, this is great for muscle building. With a lower resting heart rate you will sleep much better and that results in much more anabolism and muscle repair during that time. For it's when we rest that our muscles repair themselves.

This also means you'll be better able to deliver nutrients and oxygen to the muscles while you're training and while you're recovering because your heart is pumping more blood with each beat, which will result in more muscle growth. This also means you'll have much more energy – both to start training and to make sure those training sessions are highly productive, and allow you to exert yourself fully.

And on top of all that, jogging is still a great way to burn a lot of fat and to get a more ripped and lean physique. As much as it's not in vogue right now, it's the form of CV that was used by the famous bodybuilders Arnie, Franco Columbu and Sergio Olivia.

So guess what my advice is here once again? Combine both. Use a combination of HIIT and steady state cardio by using the former as a "finisher" at the end of a workout to burn more calories. Use the latter once a week for 4-7 miles in order to increase your cardio fitness and help you rest more.

Once again, the law of SAID means that you'll see the most extensive results as you'll adapt to both shorts spurts of exertion and longer, continuous stints. The result is the better body and the more powerful physicality.

How to Eat for Size, and Why It Really Matters!

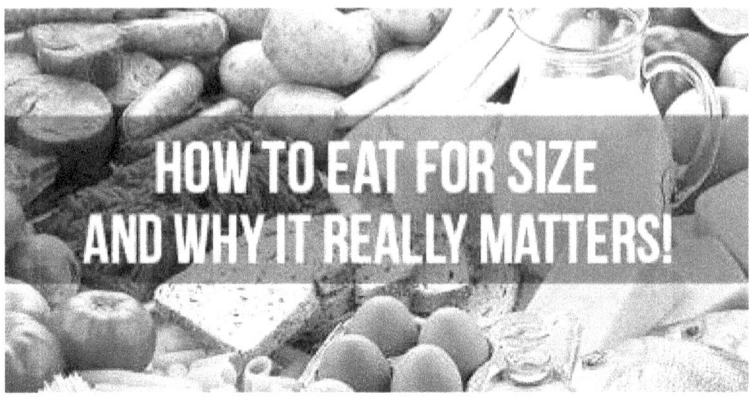

And now comes the other really important piece of that puzzle – eating for size. Because all athletes, bodybuilders and gym rats know your gains in the gym have as much to do with diet as they do your actual training… if not more so.

Remember, when you create micro tears, it is then up to your body to grow the muscle by providing it with protein and amino acids which come from your diet. If you don't have that protein, then your muscle doesn't grow. In this case, all you've done is damage the muscle and caused it pain but you haven't given it any opportunity to benefit from that stimulus. This is the epitome of "all pain, no gain".

And your diet will support you in many other ways too. If you're looking to grow, then you need to make sure you are also fueling yourself with nutrients, fats and yes, carbs.

Let's take a look at why.

Macros for Muscle Growth

If you are starting a new training regime with the goal of building muscle, then you need to also increase the amount of food you're consuming.

Most important here is the protein, for the reason we've just discussed: your muscle is made of protein. If you don't have the protein your body needs available when it needs it, then it can't grow.

So just how much protein do you need? While this is a hot topic for debate, the general consensus according to research is that you need to consume at least one gram of protein for every one pound of bodyweight. So if you weigh 170lbs, then you need to eat 170 grams of protein. That's a lot! But it's possible if you just learn to start eating lots of eggs and chicken and if you consider supplementing with protein shakes as well.

Next up is the energy. Another general consensus here is that in order to grow, you need to be maintaining a caloric surplus. That means you need to eat more calories than you burn, which makes sense when you consider that building muscle takes energy and that energy needs to come from somewhere.

Some of this energy is going to come from your protein. But the vast proportion of it will instead come from your fats and from your carbohydrates.

Fats are particularly important because they aid the absorption of other foods in your diet and because they help the body to produce testosterone, leading to better growth.

Testosterone is a sex hormone that is made from cholesterol – so you really need fat to maintain maximum anabolism.

Fat also has the benefit of releasing energy slowly and thereby not spiking the blood sugar. This is in contrast to sugar (which is found in carbs), which immediately enters the blood causing a sudden spike. This in turn causes a rise in insulin and insulin encourages fat storage. What's more, is that this then causes a blood sugar dip and that results in high cortisol which burns muscle and makes us want to snack on junk food.

So this has led some people to stop eating carbohydrates altogether. That is not the answer if you want to build muscle though. For starters, if you don't eat any carbohydrates at all (called a "ketogenic diet") then your blood will have very low sugar. This means you'll constantly be producing cortisol, which in turn will stimulate the release of something called "myostatin" – a compound that causes the breakdown of muscle tissue.

While it is possible to force your body to adapt to survive on ketone bodies (energy produced by the liver), this won't prevent catabolism or cortisol, and it won't give you as much energy for workouts and staying productive throughout the day.

So don't avoid carbs altogether, just aim to eat complex carbs that are packed with fiber (to slow the release of sugar), combine them with fats and keep them slightly more minimal.

This is what is known as calculating your macros, which in turn is short for macronutrients. The idea is that you learn how many calories you need a day (slightly more than you burn to build muscle and slightly less to lose fat) and then spread that between the three macros:

- Protein

- Fat

- Carbs

(In that order!)

Micronutrients

Then you need to make sure you are getting all of your micronutrients. These mean things like vitamins, minerals, essential fatty acids, etc. And these are really important because they make a huge difference to your body's ability to perform and to grow muscle. Vitamin C gives you more energy for example while preventing colds that can keep you out of the gym for weeks at a time. Vitamin D, zinc, magnesium and others all help encourage more testosterone production and better sleep. Vitamin B12 encourages energy. CoQ10 improves your body's energy metabolism…

You could write a gigantic list of all the ways different vitamins and minerals help you and then you could try and hunt down all those things as supplements. But much better? Just get it all in your diet.

So the biggest tip of all is to avoid empty calories. These are processed foods lie Mars Bars, Coca-Cola, crisps, etc.

These give you lots of calories without providing any valuable nutrition and they meanwhile provide a lot of sugar with no fiber or fat to slow it down.

This might sound like it wouldn't have a big impact, but trust me, you eat a nutrient rich diet and you will feel MUCH better in the gym and more able to work out. This is serious stuff!

The Importance of Rest and Recovery

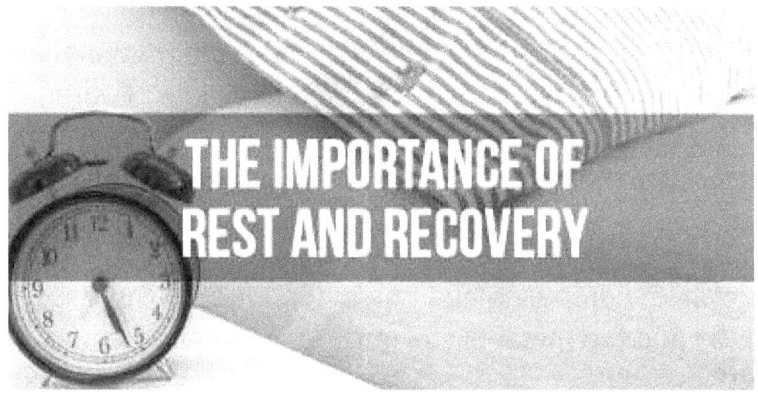

We've seen how important food it is to make sure you actually benefit from all your training and now is the time to examine something else that's majorly important: rest.

This is where a lot of guys who want to get big go wrong. They decide they want to build muscle and so to do that, they start training with great intensity and for long periods of time. That might include running, HIIT, weightlifting and more but whatever they do, they go at it 100%, so that they're dripping in sweat and close to exhaustion. Then the next day, they get up and they go at it again!

So what's happening here?

Well, during training they are breaking down muscle by creating micro tears. But instead of allowing that muscle to recover the next day, they're hitting it again even harder when it's already deteriorated. This means it can't grow and in fact will become weaker over time!

But more to the point, this kind of training takes its toll on the central nervous system. All exercise triggers the release of stress hormones because really you are putting the body under stress. When you lift weights and cause damage, your body will respond as though you're fighting or running from a predator and it will produce lots of cortisol, lots of adrenaline and lots of norepinephrine. Remember what we said about cortisol earlier: it triggers the breakdown of muscle to use for fuel!

Meanwhile, adrenaline and norepinephrine will increase fat burning and the metabolism, leading to even more muscle deterioration.

This will also hurt the sleep and eventually it can even lead to overtraining at which point the central nervous system becomes exhausted. At this point, your body has secreted as much adrenaline and as much excitatory hormones as it can – leaving you listless and prone to illness.

Training Like a Lion

So instead, your objective should be to train like a lion. That means you'll train hard, but you'll then rest hard too. When you're not training, you should be relaxing and you should be eating. Train, eat, sleep and repeat!

This also means you need to try and avoid stress, you need to maintain good sleep hygiene and you need to resist the urge to keep training with zero breaks. In fact, taking a whole week off every six to eight weeks will often be one of the best things you can do. This is called a "de-load week" and you can use it to focus on other things like flexibility or technique with light weights.

In short, if you're not seeing the growth you want and you expect… try training less, not more!

Supplementation – Your Complete Guide

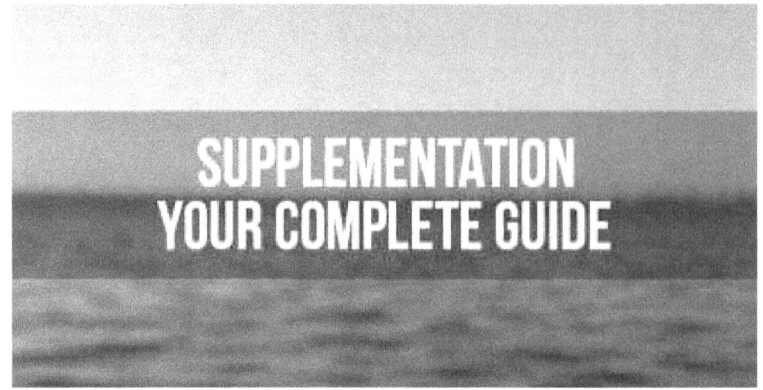

So where is supplementation going to fit into all of this? Is this something you need to be worrying about?

The answer is no, but here are a few things to consider …

Supplementation is never required. There is no single supplement that you absolutely need and you can definitely grow without any of them. But that said, there are also several that will help you to grow much more quickly if you do choose to use them.

Here are the only three that I recommend taking:

Protein Shake

Protein shake is simply protein in a highly convenient and usually tasty form. The most common form of this is whey protein, which is a type of protein that comes from milk and is removed during the cheese-making process. It's completely natural, but it offers a lean source of highly bioavailable protein.

If you can get your protein from your food alone, that's better of course. But when you're aiming for 150-200 grams of protein a day, being able to quickly mix up a shake is something of a blessing.

Protein shake does come in various forms and can contain varying amounts of calories as well as added micronutrients. While these can sometimes be helpful, normally it's best to focus on a more plain protein supplement and to get the rest from elsewhere. If you are buying them premade, watch out for added sugar.

Creatine

Creatine is a supplement that effectively allows you to convert used ATP (AMP and ADP) back into more ATP, so it can last longer. This means the muscles can use more ATP before even switching to the glycogen stores, giving you a couple seconds more exertion.

But what's also exciting about creatine is that it encourages your muscles to store more fluids. This can lead immediately to greater muscle volume if you respond well, with zero additional effort on your part! It's also very cheap.

Multivitamin

Finally, I do recommend a good multivitamin. A lot of people do not and say that they're not worth the money, but when they're well designed, they will use thoughtful combinations and timed releases to make sure your body is able to effectively absorb the nutrients therein. The existence of things like Soylent (a single supplement that contains all the nutrients you need to live off of!) shows that the body is capable of getting goodness in this form.

If you then take a product that will provide vitamin C, vitamin D, B12, zinc, magnesium and all that other good stuff, it should help to give you more energy, better sleep and better anabolism!

The Weider Principles and Other Advanced Methods for Increasing Intensity

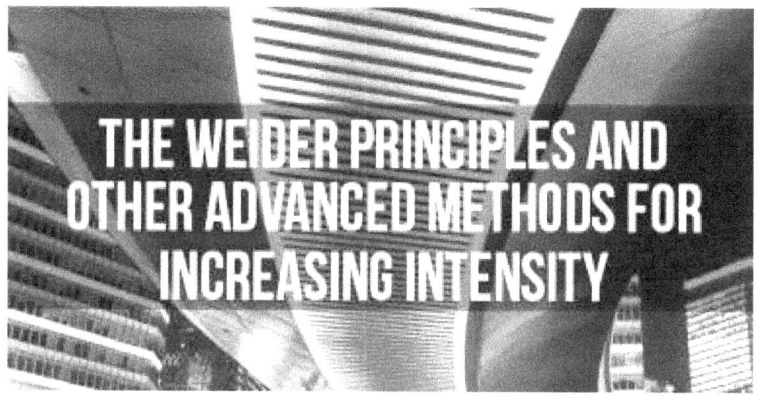

We have talked in some depth about the idea of the drop set, but now it's time to consider some of the other methods that bodybuilders have been using for a long time to push themselves harder and that powerbuilders can also adapt.

These methods are sometimes referred to as the Weider Principles, as they were catalogued by fitness media mogul and bodybuilding legend Joe Weider.

Mechanical Drop Sets and Giant Sets

Remember the drop set?

Now you're going to take this concept and run with it by introducing the idea of the mechanical drop set. In the mechanical drop set, you assume you don't have multiple weights for the same movement – or that it's not easy to swap your weights without pausing in between sets.

So what you do instead is that you move from one move onto an easier one. An example of this might be to go from one handed push-ups, to push-ups, to push-ups on your knees.

In this scenario, you're still using the same muscles predominantly, but by switching the angle or the technique, you're making it easier and allowing yourself to carry on.

You can then also use this concept to combine a powerlifting workout with a bodybuilding one, by switching from harder exercises to easier ones. This time, the example might be to go from a squat or a deadlift and then to move straight into a leg extension or a hamstring curl. You've pre-exhausted the quads and hamstrings and then you're focusing on them to brutally "finish them off".

When you combine lots of different exercises into one big set like this, we call it a giant set. And my recommendation is that you use this strategy to also combine some of the other concepts we've been looking at – such as the use of stretching, eccentric isometrics or overcoming isometrics.

You could start with overcoming isometrics at the beginning of the giant set for example and then move onto overcoming isometrics later on. In a later chapter, we'll be looking at some more techniques like these that you can throw into the mix to really create some brutal workouts.

Now it's really up to you which powerbuilding method you're going to use – but trying one of these will ensure that you are covering all bases and giving yourself the best chance of growth and strength gains.

Burns

Burns are something absolutely brutal that you can use at the end of a drop set of any kind, or even a regular set.

The idea is that you've reached failure and you can't do a single extra rep. But what you can do is half of a rep. And for that reason, you're now going to continue pumping reps but only doing half each time. You're now just bobbing the weight up and down on the spot, or bobbing your body up and down. And in doing this, you're using up every last bit of energy and really burning yourself out to nothing, tearing every last fiber! They're called burns, because they … burn!

Negatives

A negative is one way of performing a negative isometric. The idea is that you're using a weight that is too heavy to lift and so instead, you're going to get someone to help you lift it, or lift it with your other hand, and then you're just going to fight the resistance. A way you can do this on the pull up bar is to jump up and then just lower yourself as slowly as you possibly can.

Muscle Confusion

This is the concept that the muscles grow best when you keep throwing new challenges at them and they don't know what to expect. So in this case, that might mean targeting the muscle from lots of different angles, or it might mean using lots of different tempos. At the very least, this is going to maximize the different types of muscle you're using and maximize the different angles, thereby hitting a greater range of muscle fibers.

Speed training

Speed training is not a Weider principle, but rather another method that Bruce Lee used. Here, the idea is that you're simply going to lift weights as normal, except you're going to try and do so as quickly as you can. What this then does is to once again recruit the faster muscle twitch fibers. Why? Because as far as your muscle and your body is concerned, this is the exact same thing as lifting more weight. To your muscle, acceleration and resistance both require force. There's no differentiation and thus both types of movement engage the most fast twitch fibers. Jumping movements also do this and are referred to as plyometric exercises.

Instinctive Training

The eventual goal of your lifting is to get to the point where you can use purely instinctive training. This means that you know your own body so well, that you can actually feel what works and what doesn't, and you can tell when you're getting the pump, when you're creating those tiny micro tears and when you're accidentally doing damage.

This is a great point to get to because it means that you can throw the rule book out the window. Now, you can increase and decrease the challenge of your workout based purely on how it feels and you can thereby provide just the right type of challenge at any given point.

How to Stay Ripped When Getting Bigger

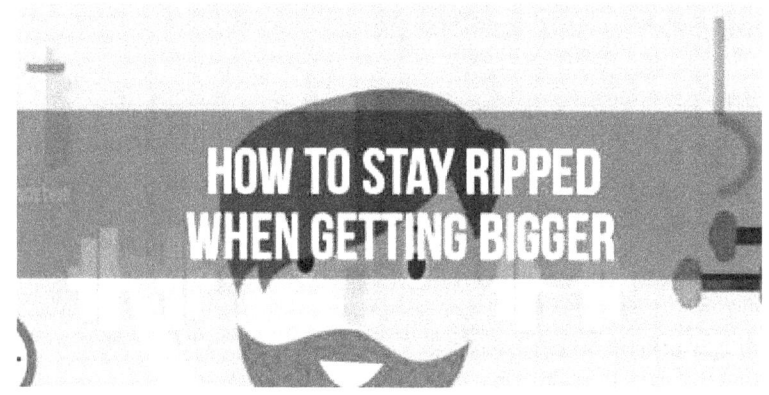

Now comes one more bodybuilding-versus-the-world question: should you bulk and cut?

For those not in the know, bulking and cutting means alternating between trying to pack on muscle (maintaining a caloric surplus and getting lots of rest) and then trying to burn off the fat (maintaining a caloric deficit and doing lots of cardio). Seeing as the methods are so different, some people believe it's impossible to do both at the same time.

But others disagree.

One argument, is that if you hover just around your daily calorie burn (you can work this out with a fitness tracker, or just by calculating your AMR), then you can slowly add muscle without adding too much fat.

Another option is to use something like intermittent fasting. This means eating normally for growth 5 days of the week and then eating a very low calorie count (about 500) for two more days of the week.

When you do this, you can reliably maintain growth, but then just cut away the excess fat and increase your insulin sensitivity two of the days. It's like bulking and cutting every week and it prevents your body from becoming too well adapted to any one type of eating.

But the problem with this is that it's a very tough way to eat and often it's also very inconvenient. You try explaining to your gran why you can't eat the delicious cake she just cooked you!

So instead, all you need to do is to do something similar, but not so extreme. That means you're going to be eating a caloric surplus some days and then going lower on other days when it suits you. This doesn't have to mean fasting at all though – it's perfectly adequate to simply eat a lower amount of calories, such as 200-300 below your AMR (active metabolic rate).

Combined with the fact that you're training both for size and power and that you're incorporating two types of cardio in as well, and you should find that this allows you to "clean bulk" while retaining your definition. This is the best way to get what is known as athletic aesthetics. That means a body that performs, but that looks the part too!

Your Complete Program for Power and Size

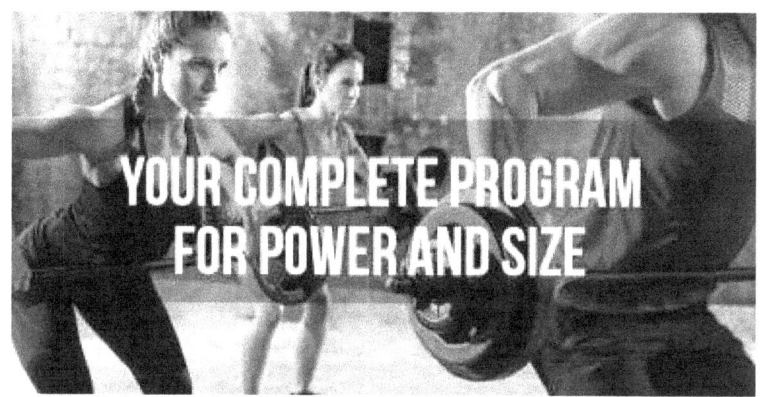

Now it's time that we bring all that together into one routine. To do that, we're going to take everything we've learned and build it into an actual program.

And for this, we need a way to separate our movements without making it impossible to use our compound movements too.

Fortunately, just such a split exists:

PPL

PPL stands for "Push, Pull, Legs" and it's the ideal routine for building a powerbuilding program around. Remember that if you go full bodybuilding, then you'll be hitting each muscle group so hard that you need to wait a week before training it again. We can't do that, but what we can do is to divide our routine into all the muscles that pull (biceps, lats, traps) and all the muscles that push (pecs, triceps, shoulders).

On these days, we'll start with compound movements that will work them all together and then we'll follow that up with isolation exercises and drop sets once they're pre-exhausted.

On the other day – L – we're going to focus on our big strength moves, which are the deadlift, the squat and things like the clean-and-press or kettlebell swing. Putting these on leg day gives us a great chance to focus on the power moves and to really stimulate some growth. In fact, we're going to perform two leg days because this is so useful! And after each of these, we'll use a 10 minute HIIT finshier.

And finally, we will do one day of steady state cardio, running 4-6 miles to improve overall fitness and burn more fat.

The Training Itself

For the training itself, you're going to be starting with bigger lifts, then moving directly into smaller/easier lifts and reducing the weight. The objective is to focus on both high weights to begin with and then increasing your time-under-tension.

Aim for a good few exercises per body part and try not to exceed 40 minutes in total.

A sample push day then, might start with bench press with a high weight, going straight into a drop set. You might then set up a mechanical drop set going from bench press, to clapping press-ups, to press-ups. After repeating that three times, you might perform burns on the last set. Finally, you might move on to dumbbell flies with a very slow negative portion of the movement.

Then, you would probably try doing something similar for the shoulders and then the triceps, before calling it a day.

The Diet

For our diet, our aim is to consume 1 gram of protein for every 1 pound of body weight. We're going to reduce carbohydrates and aim for complex carbs, but we're not going to avoid them altogether. Five days of the week we'll be aiming to consume slightly more carbohydrates than we burn off (about 200) and two days of the week we'll go for a calorie deficit (about 200) – we can alter this though dependent on how our body seems to be responding.

Also very important is that we're going to be aiming to make sure all of this food is highly nutritious and packed with nutrients. If you're struggling to stick to this diet, my tip is to try and eat your healthiest meals for breakfast and lunch. These tend to be the less social meals and they also tend to be more routine. Find a good breakfast you like and maybe a good salad bar for lunch and keep it consistent!

Conclusions and Recap

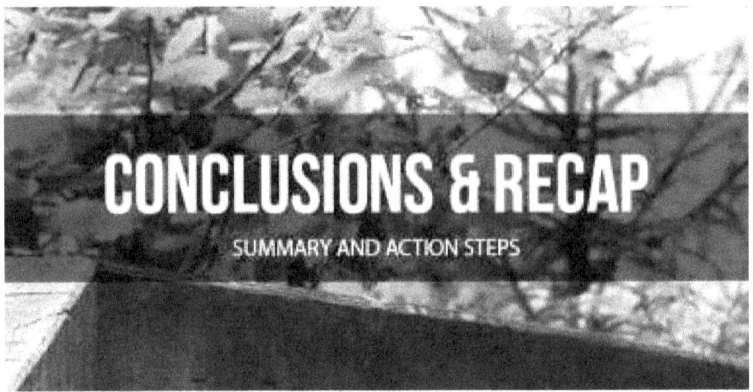

Using this program, you should find that no matter your body type, you start to see some progress. Then, when you really know what's working for you and what your goals are, you can hone your approach to be more specifically tailored to you.

But along the way, you'll have learned that there are a lot of ways to approach a training program and that these can trigger drastically different results depending on your body type and on your goals. We've learned the value of lifting weights slow sometimes. We've seen the power of using heavier weights. We've discovered the role of the mind. And we've seen why diet plays such a big part in it all.

Hopefully, now you understand the science behind the hypertrophy, you'll be better able to craft a program that works wonders for you and you'll have more knowledge to help you experiment with different approaches.

And just maybe, you'll also have gained more appreciation for power building – a highly effective form of training no matter your goals.

Good luck and may your training journey be a fruitful one!

Checklist

Want to understand the mechanisms of hypertrophy so that you can stimulate the maximum increase in muscle growth and strength through your training?

This checklist will help you to do just that by providing you with all of the information we saw in the book, condensed into some simple steps and points that you can follow...

Types of Hypertrophy

There are two types of hypertrophy according to many thinkers on the subject matter. These are:

Sarcoplasmic hypertrophy

Myofibrillar hypertrophy

Myofibrillar hypertrophy means that the muscle fibers are tearing as a result of intense exercise, which in turn encourages the body to repair them with amino acids subsequently. This allows those fibers to grow back stronger and thicker, thereby making the muscles themselves stronger and thicker.

Sarcoplasmic hypertrophy on the other hand involves increasing the sarcoplasm in the muscles to increase muscle endurance.

So how do you train each?

To train for sarcoplasmic hypertrophy you train using longer sets with more repetitions and you use lighter weights.

To train for myofibrillar hypertrophy you train with heavier weights and use this for fewer repetitions.

There are also some additional techniques and methods you can take into account. For example:

You can create a better "mind muscle connection" by training with heavier weights and by concentrating more on the muscle during training to really feel the contraction.

You can also do the same thing by using "overcoming isometrics"

The type of training you use will affect which muscle fibers the body recruits. You have two types:

- Fast twitch muscle fiber – for explosive movements and bursts of energy

- Slow twitch muscle fiber – for continuous exercises and multiple repetitions

- Heavier training recruits more fast twitch fiber, so too does faster training

- Tension under stretch using eccentric isometrics is another way to cause more micro tears and muscle damage

- Sarcoplasmic hypertrophy involves maximum metabolic stress achieved through the longest time under tension.

- Your objective then is to choose whether you want to train more for size or more for power and then to use the appropriate training.

What's also useful here though, is to recognize that different body types respond to different types of training. You might have a higher density of slow twitch muscle fiber for instance, or you might have a slow metabolism.

Introducing Powerbuilding

This is where powerbuilding comes in. This is a form of training that combines traditional bodybuilding-type training with powerlifting-style training. The aim is to increase size and strength, function and form.

To do this, you can combine the exercises we've seen in numerous ways:

- Have a couple of days training with powerlifting moves and a couple of days training with bodybuilding moves

- Train with powerlifting moves at the start of a workout and then move to more isolation, bodybuilding techniques toward the end.

- Use training techniques like drop sets that allow you to combine both heavy exercises and longer time under tension.

Eating Right

You also need to combine this training with the right diet. The easiest way to understand the right approach to diet is simply to look at the various different rules you need to try and understand:

- To build muscle, you should be in a caloric surplus meaning you eat more calories than you burn off

- To lose weight, you should be in a caloric deficit, meaning you burn more calories than you eat

- To build muscle, you need to be consuming 1 gram of protein for every 1 pound of body weight

You also need to consider your other macros. Fats are important as a slow release energy source. Carbs are important to prevent your blood sugar crashing, which releases cortisol and myostatin.

Calculate your AMR (active metabolic rate) to know how many calories you burn in a day.

Then calculate your macros by working how many calories you should be getting from each food group:

- **Protein**

- **Carbs**

- **Fats**

Try to eat a nutrient dense diet. This means you should be consuming foods high in vitamins and minerals.

No supplements are completely necessary but the three most useful ones are:

- **Protein shake**

- **Creatine**

- **Some kind of multivitamin**

Give all this a try and prepare to see some impressive results in your training!

Your Hypertrophy Resource Sheet

Now that you've read the full book, you should have a good idea of how to build muscle strength and size and you should understand the actual science that goes on behind the scenes and that leads to hypertrophy.

All that's left is to start putting that into action. This resource sheet will make that all the easier by providing you with the information, resources, terminology and more – all easily accessible for you to dip into as you need.

Diet

Let's start with the diet. In order to build big muscle, you need to make sure you are providing your body with the protein and calories it needs, while losing weight means keeping your calorie intake lower than the amount you burn in a given day.

In both scenarios, you need to make sure that you know your AMR which is your Active Metabolic Rate. You can calculate this by using the following math:

First, you calculate your BMR which is your Basal Metabolic Rate – the amount of calories you're likely to burn based on your height, age, weight, etc.

Men:

BMR = 66 + (6.23 x weight in pounds) + (12.7 x height in inches) – (6.8 x age in years)

Women:

BMR = 655 + (4.35 x weight in pounds) + (4.7 x height in

inches) – (4.7 x age in years)

Now take the score for your BMR and multiply it by:

- 1.2 if you're sedentary (little or no exercise)

- 1.375 if you're lightly active (you exercise 1-3 times a week)

- 1.55 if you're moderately active (you exercise or work about average)

- 1.725 if you're very active (you train hard for 6-7 days a week)

- 1.9 if you're highly active (you're a physical laborer or a professional athlete)

From here, you can then calculate your macros. Remember, your macros are your:

- Carbs

- Protein

- Fats

You need to eat:

1 gram of protein for every 1 pound of bodyweight.

Now use this calculator to work out the rest:
http://www.bodybuilding.com/fun/macronutrients_calculator.htm

You'll also need to track those macronutrients. The way most people do this is with the free calorie calculator and diet tracker My Fitness Pal. You can find this here: https://www.myfitnesspal.com/

You can also track the number of calories you are burning any given day more accurately by using a fitness tracker. One of the best ones is the Microsoft Band 2, which you can find here: https://www.microsoft.com/microsoft-band/

The Routine

For the routine itself, you need to decide what your goals are and your training philosophy. You can learn more about that here:

https://www.t-nation.com/training/developing-a-training-philosophy

You can then also take a look at the different schools of training and how they operate. Here are some primers on different types of training:

Powerbuilding:
http://www.myprotein.com/thezone/training/powerbuilding-strength-size-definition-training-splits-workout-routines/

CrossFit: http://www.crossfit.com

Bodybuilding: http://www.bodybuilding.com

Powerlifting: http://www.powerlifting-ipf.com/

MovNat: https://www.movnat.com/

Functional Training:
http://www.humankinetics.com/excerpts/excerpts/what-is-functional-training

Calisthenics: http://ashotofadrenaline.net/calisthenics-workout-plan/

Each of these training methods is different, but they are all also perfectly valid. You simply have to find the type of training right for your particular goals.

Of course you then also need to find the best type of exercises you can utilize in combination with your chosen discipline. You can do this by looking up a range of different indexes and catalogues of exercises. One of the best of these can be found at bodybuilding.com:
http://www.bodybuilding.com/exercises/list/index/selected/a

Inspiration and Community

Also handy at bodybuilding.com is the excellent Bodyspace (**http://bodyspace.bodybuilding.com**). This is a social network that works very similarly to something like Facebook, except it is entirely based around fitness and working out. This means that you can post your images to get critiqued, or you can engage in active discussions.

Some other great websites for learning more about bodybuilding and strengthen training are Breaking Muscle (**http://www.breakingmuscle.com**) and T-Nation (**http://www.t-nation.com**). Both of these sites provide a slightly more interesting type of content that includes lots of detailed information about the science of hypertrophy and anabolism.

As you've probably guessed at this point, Bodybuilding.com is generally a fantastic resource for learning about bodybuilding and for finding different exercises, different training regimes etc.

For something a little different, check out Tim Ferriss' blog *The 4 Hour Blog*. It digs deep into ways you can hack hypertrophy and stimulate growth with a MED or Minimum Effective Dose.

You can also find some great inspiration and tips on YouTube. Some of the best channels include:

AthleanX – Jeff Cavaliere helped to make "athletic aesthetics" cool before anyone else was even using the term. Jeff teaches you how to train like an athlete and provides a lot of very functional instruction about how to lift correctly etc.

BodybuildingRev – This is a German YouTube channel but most of the content is either available in English or with English subtitles. Either way, it's worth watching because it has some very interesting videos that showcase the different types of training. These include strength wars where a bodybuilder might face off against a fitness model or a CrossFit champion for example.

Bodybuilding.com – Bodybuilding.com also has a great YouTube channel that features many workouts, lots of diet plans etc.

Supplements

Finally, consider the following supplements as useful additions to your training if you want to get a slight edge:

- **Protein Shake**: A whey protein shake will fuel the body with the raw amino acids it needs to build more muscle. This makes it much more convenient to get hold of that kind of protein, without having to spend a lot of money or cook up meals. Note that you can also get additional types of protein shake:

  - **Casein** – A slow release protein, also made from milk

  - **Egg**

- **Soy** – A vegetarian friendly protein that isn't as bioavailable and may raise oestrogen levels

- **Creatine**: Creatine can give you an energy boost in the gym but as a free added bonus, it also encourages the muscles to retain more fluid. This can instantly result in great muscle size!

- **Multivitamin and Mineral Tablet**: These can give you an edge by making sure you are getting all of those crucial vitamins and minerals to help fuel muscle growth, provide you with more energy in your workouts and generally make you more effective in your training.

Other Fitness Books by This Author

If you would like to read more relative books from this author, here is a list of the <u>CreateSpace links, titles and descriptions:</u>

<u>https://www.createspace.com/6114822</u>

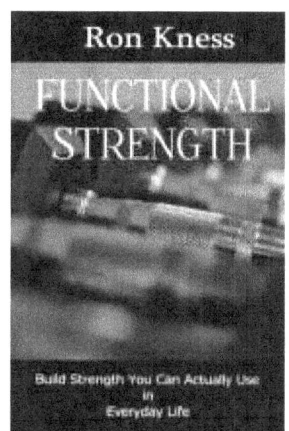

Health and fitness fads come and go all the time but unfortunately not all of them are worth your time and effort. Some of them don't work, some of them are over-hyped and some of them are just plain dangerous.

But 'functional strength' is different. While functional strength is very much in vogue right now, it's not a 'fad' by any means. In fact, functional strength is the opposite of a fad and it's a step in the right direction for all of fitness.

That's because functional strength take it all back: takes it all back to the reasons that most of us started training in the first place. Or at least the reasons we should be training.

When you train for functional strength and fitness, everything becomes easier: from opening a jam jar, to helping a friend move furniture, to getting out of bed in the morning.

And if you want to train for your appearance as your first priority? Well then this is still the right way to go: because when you train for strength and power, you look much better.

Don't believe me?

Then think about it logically: the reason that humans find healthy people attractive is because we assume they have better genetics and are better able to protect themselves and their families. Someone with functional strength really can do all those things and really is healthier – so they send all of those unconscious signals that make them more attractive to the opposite sex!

Learn how to build strength that will not only improve everyday life, but also your appearance.

https://www.createspace.com/4961770

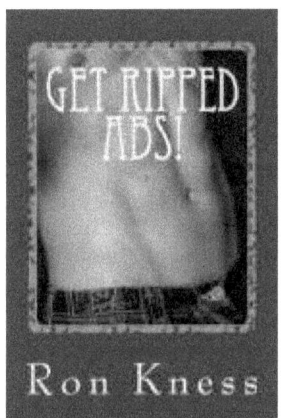

We are enthralled with six-pack abs. In the fitness world, having a set seems to be the ultimate visual evidence of a fit body. People go to great lengths to try and get "washboard" abs, but few succeed. Why is that?

The truth is we all have the same abdominal muscles, so if fact we all have six-pack abs. But having them and being able to see them can be two very different things.

The focus of this book is to show you what you can do with your abs to work them, define them and make them come through visually, so that when you rip off your shirt, people take notice.

Covered in the book is first how to get rid of the belly fat covering your abs through diet and cardio training. Then it moves into an exercise routine that will start to define your abs. Finally maintenance is addressed - once you have ripped abs, what you can do to keep them.

https://www.createspace.com/5520238

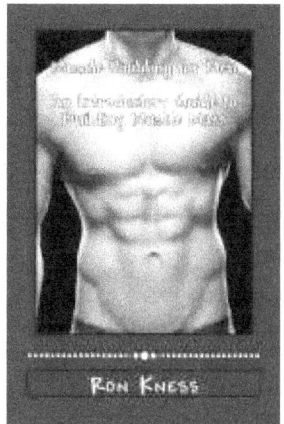

In my book Muscle Building for Men – An Introductory Guide to Building Muscle Mass, I reveal a successful method of building muscle.

Your best bet is to formulate an all-over workout routine that helps you do three things:
• Burn fat
• Build muscle mass
• Strengthen your muscle

Burn Fat

Burning off fat is really a quite simple process. All you have to do is burn mor3e calories than you take in. In fact you have to burn 3,500 more calories per week than you take in to lose one pound of weight. One of the best ways to burn fat is through cardio-type exercises, such as running, biking or playing any sport that keeps you moving all the time and gets both your heart rate and breathing up into the fat burning zones – a target rate that is 80% of 220 minus your age.

Build Muscle Mass

While cardio burns off excess calories and the fat and weight associated with it, the only way to build muscle is through weight or strength training. Working with light weights but numerous repetitions will tone and tighten muscles for a well-defined look, but if you want to actually build muscle mass, you have to lift heavier weights, but fewer repetitions.

Strengthen your Muscle

While getting leaner by burning off fat and building muscle mass are two ways to help strengthen your muscles, what we are talking about here is healthy eating. Without a proper diet, the other two will be harder to achieve. Part of losing weight and getting stronger is not only burning more calories, but taking in less calories to begin with.

What many people new to muscle building don't understand is that you actually are going to eat more food, but consume fewer calories. The key is to eat the right kinds of food; foods that will fuel your fat loss, build muscle and overall strengthen your muscles.

https://www.createspace.com/6096909

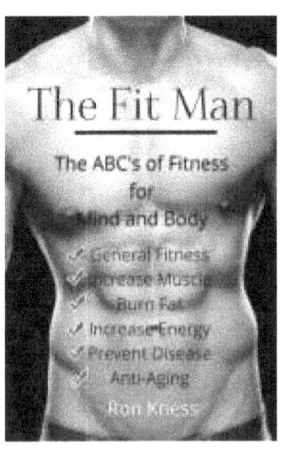

If you're completely new to working out, you will soon become amazed by the changes your body is capable of and hopefully become an avid iron enthusiast.

The truth is, we all desire a good body. Moreover, it comes with many perks, far beyond what you see when you look at a chiseled six-pack and bulging arms. If done safely, you've just added years to your life!

Training shouldn't be rocket science - when it boils down to it, your body knows what it needs. Do not become a victim of "analysis paralysis" trying every new routine that comes out!

Stick to the basics of performing full body, or exercises that utilize more than one muscle group and you will develop true functional fitness (those movements that translate well to the things you do every day in real life).

The Fit Man can help you stay fit and healthy for many years to come.

About the Author

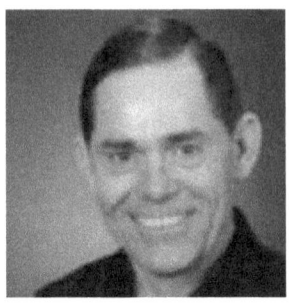

I grew up in Central Minnesota, where my parents owned and operated a fishing resort. Once out of high school I tried a couple of semesters of college, only to quit halfway through the Spring term; I decided at that time that college wasn't for me.

Then I decided to follow my father's previous occupation as an auto mechanic. I graduated from a two-year of vocational training course and worked as a mechanic for five years. While in vocational training, I decided to join the National Guard where I eventually ended up working full-time for 32 years.

So how does all of this relate to writing? In one of my leadership schools, the instructor, who was an English teacher at a juvenile detention center, presented writing to me in a whole new way - a way that started to develop my interest in working with words.

I eventually went back to college on the GI Bill while I was working and earned my Bachelor's degree in Business Administration. Taking a class or two per semester at night and on weekends took me seven years to complete my degree.

Fast forward about 40 years and I now have published over 75 books on Amazon for Kindle, CreateSpace and other publishing platforms.

Besides my own writing, I also ghostwrite ebooks, reports, articles, blogs and do Kindle conversions for clients on a variety of topics.

Today my wife and I are retired from our careers and live in Gold Canyon, AZ. I now write as a retirement business where you'll find me happily sitting in my office typing away on my laptop as I work on my next book or ghostwriting project . . . that is if we are not traveling on a cruise ship - our new-found mode of travel.

www.ingramcontent.com/pod-product-compliance
Lightning Source LLC
Chambersburg PA
CBHW070123290526

45789CB00005B/2126